TEA TREE OIL

(Melaleuca alternifolia)

BY DEANNE TENNEY

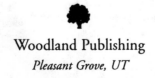

Woodland Publishing
Pleasant Grove, UT

The information in this booklet is for educational purposes only. It is not intended to be used to diagnose any ailment or prescribe any remedy. It should not be substituted for professional medical help. An individual should consult a duly approved health professional for any condition which requires their services. Neither the author nor publisher directly or indirectly dispense medical advice or prescribe the use of natural remedies as a form of treatment.

CONTENTS

INTRODUCTION 5

HISTORY 6

HARVESTING AND PRODUCTION . . 8

RESEARCH 9

Compounds Found in Tea Tree Oil . 10
Toxicity 11
Antiseptic Properties . . . 12
Drug-Resistant Strains . . . 13
A Strong Bactericide . . . 16
Fungal Diseases 17
Yeast Infections 17
A Mild Anesthetic . . . 19
Help for Acne 19
A Natural Insecticide . . . 21
An Immune System Builder . . 22

TEA TREE OIL SUPPLEMENTS . . 24

USES OF TEA TREE OIL . . . 24

ENDNOTES 31

INTRODUCTION

Tea tree oil is extracted from the leaves of *Melaleuca alternifolia,* a shrub-like tree found in the northeast tropical coastal region of New South Wales and Queensland, Australia. There are over 300 different varieties of tea tree but only a few are known to produce the valuable medicinal oil, and other species are being studied to see if they contain any of the beneficial properties of tea tree oil. The Melaleuca alternifolia tree is usually cultivated for extracting the valuable oil on plantations in Australia.

Tea tree oil has been used to treat many different conditions. Some include athlete's foot, acne, boils, burns, warts, vaginal infections, tonsillitis, sinus infections, ringworm, skin rashes, impetigo, herpes, corns, head lice, cold sores, canker sores, insect bites and fungal infections. It is truly a remarkable oil with valuable properties for healing. It can be found in toothpaste, cosmetics, shampoos, conditioners, deodorants, sunscreens, insect repellents, bath oils, acne treatments, creams, lotions, soaps and many other products.

The amazing thing about tea tree oil is that it is one of the most effective essential oils. It is found in almost all the pharmacies in Australia and is used extensively. It contains antibacterial properties as well as antifungal properties. Tea tree oil is considered a non-poisonous, non-irritating antiseptic with very strong properties. It is considered safe and effective and can be used for extended periods of time without complication.

THE HISTORY OF TEA TREE OIL

The Bundjalung aborigines in New South Wales, Australia have long known the value of the tea tree's crushed leaves. They were known to chew on the leaves to help heal a cold or other disorders. It was used as a medicinal agent for cuts, burns, bites, infected wounds, and many skin ailments. They drank a tea from made from the crushed leaves for just about any sickness. They inhaled the crushed leaves to treat respiratory ailments. They also bathed in the waters near where the trees grow. These waters were thought to have healing properties because of the close proximity to the trees.[1]

Captain James Cook

Tea tree oil caught the attention of Captain James Cook, a lieutenant with the British Royal Navy, on his second trip to Australia in 1770, an expedition with botanist Sir John Banks, who collected samples of the leaves and took them back to England for further study. Captain Cook became interested after watching the aborigines make tea from the crushed leaves of the tree and use it to treat different ailments. Captain Cook and his sailors made a tea from the leaves and enjoyed the spicy, pleasant aroma and flavor. They called it "tea tree" after making the tea. A tea was also made using the leaves by the early settlers who followed the example of the Aborigines. These settlers relied on the leaves to cure many ailments.

The Early 1900s

Many dentists and surgeons relied on tea tree oil during the 1920s as a disinfectant for wounds and incisions. They found it to be remarkably effective in preventing infections from occurring. It was regularly used by dentists for treating various conditions such as gingivitis, periodontal disease, infections and bleeding gums. Physicians prescribed tea tree oil for cystitis, yeast infections. fungal infections, skin ailments and throat infections.[2]

World War II

During World War II, tea tree oil was mixed with machine oil during wartime production in Australia. It helped protect the workers against infection caused by cuts and scrapes which occured when coming in contact with metal filings. It was effective in preventing dangerous infections.

They also used tea tree oil as a disinfectant. It was included in the first aid kits of the medics for medical treatment during battle. The oil was poured directly into wounds as soon as possible to protect from infection. It was thought of as one of the most important ingredients in the first aid kit. The oil was so valuable that its production was thought of as essential during World War II. The producers of the oil were exempt from military service because of the need of the oil during the war.

After World War II, the use and production of tea tree oil was limited. This may have been due to the general trend toward synthetic medication and antibiotics that swept the modern world. Synthetic preparations were cheap and easy to prepare. And many thought these advancements in medical science were superior to old treatments used in the past.

Now many are rediscovering the value of tea tree oil. Its healing properties are becoming recognized in the United States and Europe as well as Australia. Its significance in healing may benefit many individuals for years to come.

HARVESTING AND PRODUCTION

The Melaleuca alternifolia tree is found naturally in swampy, lowland areas around the Clarence and Richmond River territories in Australia. Many of the plants grow and thrive naturally in this area because of the tropical climate. The trees have long trunks and branches. They usually grow to less than twenty feet in height. The leaves are bright green and feathery in appearance and sometimes have yellow, clustering flowers. The leaves grow on top and when trimmed, revive within eighteen months to thick foliage. Small companies used to produce the oil traveling into the wooded areas and cutting the branches of the trees. Now, because of an increase in demand, major producers have developed tree farms to extract the oil. The leaves are cut twice a year allowing the trees to grow and thrive. The cropping seems to help stimulate regrowth of the branches and promote healthy trees.[3]

Cutting the leaves can be an adventure in itself. The trees are found naturally in remote, swampy areas that are hard to reach. The branches must be cut with machetes. The foliage is dense around the areas where the trees grown, which makes it difficult to harvest. Plantations growing and harvesting the leaves have added to increased production for the benefit of all areas of the world. They are able to produce larger quantities because of the easier access and harvesting techniques.

The tree leaves are distilled to produce an almost colorless oil with a distinctive aroma similar to eucalyptus or camphor. It has a spicy, strong odor but is quite pleasant.

RESEARCH

Studies done on the oil have shown that the pure tea tree oil is an extremely complex substance. In 1922 the first known scientific research was done on the properties of tea tree oil. Arthur R. Penfold, an Australian government chemist, found that tea tree oil is a powerful antiseptic. In fact, he found it to be 12 times more effective than phenol (carbolic acid) which was the most powerful antiseptic at the time without doing any damage to the skin. He presented his findings to the Royal Society of New South Wales and England.

Later, a paper was published in the *Medical Journal of Australia* in 1930 discussing the great benefits of tea tree oil including its non-toxicity and germicidal properties. By 1937 it was regarded as beneficial for healing infections with pus and of the blood.

Tea tree oil contains at least 48 different organic compounds, and not all of the elements have been identified. The compounds work together to produce the healing abilities found in the oil. Single elements do not have the same healing benefits. Tea tree oil in its pure form is a natural combination to heal and soothe. The compounds consist mainly of terpinenes, cymones, pinenes, terpineols, cineol, sesquiterpenes, and sesquiterpene alcohols. It also contains the organic compound virdiflorene. The elements in tea tree oil are being researched to determine which combination of the compounds works best together and in what amounts.

Research done in the 1950s and early 1960s found that tea tree oil is a germicide and fungicide with additional characteristics of dissolving pus and debris.[4] Recent studies have found it effective for thrush, vaginal infections of candida albicans, staph infections, athlete's foot, hair and scalp problems, mouth sores, muscle and joint pain, and boils.[5]

Compounds Found in Tea Tree Oil

Research has found that tea tree oil is a very complex substance containing 48 different compounds. All these work together synergistically to produce the maximum healing power. These compounds consist mainly of terpinenes, cymones, pinenes, terpineols, cinerol, sesquiterpenes, and sesquiterpene alcohols.

"Tea tree leaves contain about 2 percent of a pale lemon-tinted volatile oil with a pleasant nutmeg odor. It is obtained from the leaves by steam distillation. About one-third of the oil is comprised of various terpene hydrocarbons (pinene, terpinene, cymeme); the remainder consists largely of oxygenated terpenes, particularly terpinen-4-ol, which may constitute up to 60 percent of the total oil.

Sesquiterpene hydrocarbons and oxygenated sesquiter-penes are also present."[6]

Toxicity

The Australian tea tree oil has been found to be highly effective in treating infections and destroying microbes while not irritating the skin. Many antiseptics can cause skin irritation, but tea tree oil seems to cause no harm to skin tissue.

Tea tree oil is an antiseptic and should not be taken internally. Some evidence has suggested mild organ damage from internal use. The oil, when absorbed through the skin, is non-toxic.

"There are no deaths on record from internal use or accidental overdose. However, the oil has only been proven safe for external usage. While tea tree oil cannot be regarded as being highly toxic, evidence exists that consumption may lead to internal organ damage. However, the LD 50, the standard method used to measure fatal toxicity, exceeds 30 milliliters. That means that 30 milliliters per day proved fatal to test animals. Small amounts, as in those that might be absorbed as a result of external applications, are non-toxic. Further evidence for its low toxicity is found in the fact that tea tree oils used as a carrier for natural flavors; for instance, nutmeg oil."[7]

Tea tree oil is most often recommended for exposed surfaces of the body such as the skin tissue and the mucous membranes. It should be noted that the original Australian aborigines made tea from the leaves without adverse affects. And the early settlers followed their example with positive results. But the tea was a very diluted form and the distilled oil is much stronger.

Antiseptic Properties

Tea tree oil is a complex, natural substance with potent medicinal properties. The components work synergistically in producing therapeutic results. Infectious diseases are on the rise. And tragically, many new strains are emerging that are drug resistant. Viruses are able to mutate and change shape which makes them very difficult to kill. Infections are the leading cause of visits to the doctor's office. Epidemics of influenza occur each year.

Tea tree oil can be used on fungal infections such as athlete's foot , ringworm and diaper rash. It can be applied directly to the infection several times a day. Tea tree oil is also used for dental treatment of conditions such as pyorrhea and gingivitis. It can also be applied to wounds to help in the healing process. One amazing ability of the tea tree oil is that of killing the candida yeast bacteria. It also can be used to treat many skin fungi. One problem with using antibiotics is that it allows the yeast bacteria to thrive. Using tea tree oil allows for treatment without negative side effects.

Dr. Andrew Weil says, "Tea Tree Oil is the best treatment I know for fungal infections of the skin (athlete's foot, ringworm, jock itch). It will also clear up fungal infections of the toenails or fingernails, a condition notoriously resistant to treatment, even by strong systemic antibiotics. You just paint the oil on affected areas two or three times a day."[8]

Tea tree oil is a valuable antiseptic for skin infections. It is able to penetrate the epidermis to heal from within. Clinical studies have found that tea tree oil can heal quickly and with less scarring than other treatments. The oil is even effective against *Staphylococcus aureus,* which is often difficult to treat. The oil can be applied two to three times a day with full strength. If an irritation occurs, a diluted solution can be tried. Highly diluted concentrations have been found to heal in clinical studies.

Drug-Resistant Strains

Life-threatening, obscure illness have emerged throughout the world causing panic and concern in African villages as well as in suburban communities in the United States. With world travel common place, germs are easily transported from nation to nation across miles of ocean or land. A strep bacteria resistant to antibiotics, the hantavirus, hepatitis and tuberculosis are some of the new and reemerging plagues. Hospital settings are not exempt from contamination. There are extremely serious infections contracted in hospitals each year throughout the world in the most respected hospitals. These infections are known to cause many deaths among patients, especially the elderly and those with weak immune systems.

Medical researchers now believe that this is just the beginning. They think that a new, even more serious germ will emerge. Someday, another great plague will probably appear though no one can predict where or what it will be. Infectious disease was considered to be under control with the development of drugs and antibiotics. Experts now believe that the problem is becoming astronomical. The variety of disease is increasing and the germs are extremely resilient.

Bacteria are able to develop a resistance to antibiotics. The problem stems from individuals going to the doctor and wanting a cure. They don't feel the visit was worthwhile if they don't leave with a prescription for antibiotics. A prime time news show did a study on this problem. They sent a well woman to four different doctors asking for antibiotics because of a sore throat and cold. Three of the four doctors gave her the prescription even though there appeared to be no problem at all. One doctor justified her prescription by saying that she felt in order to keep patients she needed to give them what they want. Well, an overuse of antibiotics has resulted in the ability of many bacterias to become resistant to the cure. Also individuals who are on antibiotics need to take the full course in order to kill all the bacteria responsible for the infection. If not, the strongest will survive with the ability to resist future antibiotic treatment. Increasingly, researchers are being confronted with microbes that have learned to become resistant to drugs. One example is that forty years ago gonorrhea could easily be treated with small doses of penicillin. Now it requires massive doses to kill the organism. Antibiotics should be used only as a last resort.

Streptococcus bacteria, which causes strep throat, is a very serious form that can be fatal. It is thought by some to be a return of a bacteria that causes scarlet fever, which a century ago caused thousand of deaths and then disappeared. Infections appear to occur in cycles. It can cause a drop in blood pressure as well as organ failure. It also is responsible for the cases of necrotizing fasciitis, a secondary infection that eats away at the muscle, fat, and flesh. The seriousness lies in its quick progression. The infection can spread as rapidly as one inch per hour.

Toxins released by the strep bacteria poison the skin and surrounding muscle tissue along with internal organs. This causes the immune system to quickly fail. This is similar to the way the hantavirus produces a toxin that rapidly breaks down capillary walls in the lungs causing its victims to drown in their own fluids.

If caught early enough, it can be treated with penicillin. Fortunately, this is not an antibiotic resistant strain of bacteria. If tissues has died, antibiotic therapy has no way to treat the area because blood flow has ceased. Sometimes surgery is required to remove large pieces of affected tissue and even amputation of affected limbs. These infectious microorganisms are spread primarily through open wounds or cuts in the skin. The fatality rate is approximately 28 percent among those who contract the flesh eating symptoms.

How can tea tree oil help? Tea tree oil itself consists of a complex structure which is difficult to build a resistance to. It would be extremely difficult, if not impossible, for a microbe to become resistant to the oil because of the complexity of the chemical structure. In contrast, many synthetic antibiotics contain only a single component or a simple structure. It is much easier for the microbes to figure and learn to resist these synthetically engineered products. Tea tree oil is non-toxic. It can be applied locally to an affected area and does not cause damage to the local tissue while it is able to kill on contact.

Organisms against which tea tree oil has been shown to be effective include:

- aspergillus
- Candida
- cryptosporidium
- E. Coli
- epidermophyton
- gonococcus
- herpes viruses
- microsporium
- proteus
- spirochetes
- strep
- trichophyton[9]

- baceroides
- clostridium
- diptheroids
- enterobacter
- fusobacterium
- hemophilus
- meningococcus
- petococcus
- pseudomonas
- staph
- trichinosis

A Strong Bactericide

Tea tree oil is an effective bactericide. It is safe for healthy tissue. It is a strong organic solvent and will help heal and disperse pus in pimples and wounds. It has been used to neutralize the venom of minor insect bites. It is able to kill bacteria by penetrating the skin layers and reaching deep into abscesses in the gums and even beneath the fingernails. It has been found to have some of the strongest antimicrobial properties ever discovered in a plant.[10] Essential oils all contain antiseptic and bactericidal properties in different proportions. Robert Tisserand believes tea tree oil to be specific to streptococcus, gonococcus, and pneumococcus.[11]

An extract of tea tree oil has been found effective in treating conditions such as trichomoniasis, candidiasis and cervicitis. It is used as a one percent solution in a daily douche combined with saturated tampons. No negative reactions occurred among the patients studied but the treatment was very soothing and healing.[12]

Fungal Diseases

There are thousands of different fungal diseases though only a portion of these afflict the world population. Most medical professionals believe that the incidence of these diseases is on the increase. Different types of fungi can invade almost every body tissue. And they can afflict anyone at any age. Some believe that the fungi are involved in impairing immunity. Fungal infections burden the immune system. Many fungal diseases are resistant to treatment because only the first layer of the infection is treated.

Tea tree oil is beneficial because it can penetrate deep into the skin tissues. Areas such as the skin, gums, nails and mucous membranes can be treated with the oil. It can help treat by reaching the root of the problem and even help with resistant, chronic fungal infections.

Yeast Infections

Dr. Eduardo F. Pena, M.D., studied Melaleuca alternifolia oil for its value in treating vaginitis and candida albicans. The women were treated with an emulsified 40 percent solution of the oil and 13 percent isopropyl alcohol.

"The study was conducted on 130 women suffering from four types of vaginal infections: 96 cases of trichomonal vaginitis, several cases of thrush and cervicitis, and a control group of 50 women who were treated with anti-trichoma suppositories. Out of 130 patients, all treatment was successful and the Tea Tree Oil treatments had similar results to the control group. In the 96 cases of trichomonal vaginitis, clinical cures were obtained by inserting a tampon saturated with a 1 percent solution of Melaleuca alternifolia oil which was then removed after twenty-four hours. Daily vaginal douches of 1 percent solution in one quart of water were also recommended. The number of office treatments necessary to achieve a clinical cure averaged 6, while the total number of douches per patient averaged 42. Patients commented on its pine odor and its soothing, cooling effect. It was also apparent that at no time did the patient experience irritation or burning. The clinical study indicated that tea tree oil is a penetrating germicide and fungicide with additional characteristics of dissolving pus and debris.[13]

Candida albicans has been heavily researched. It is extremely potent and hard to eradicate once it takes hold in an individual. Immune stimulation may be the best method of treating the condition. Candida infections will not develop in healthy individuals with strong immune function. Even when they are exposed, the infection will not develop. "In studying Candida researchers have gone to the extreme of infecting healthy volunteers with the organism. The yeasts proceeded to invade the bloodstream and internal organs. Then they were cultured from these regions. However, within a matter of hours yeasts could no longer be cultured, indicating that the immune systems of these individuals efficiently cleared the organisms from the tissues. Unfortunately, in today's era a great many people are afflicted with compromised immune function. What's more, even the healthiest of immune systems may find the battle overwhelming, especially if mass innoculation occurs."[14]

Tea tree oil can destroy Candida. It can penetrate deep to reach the area of infection. Application should continue for a period of time to ensure the destruction of the infection. Tampons saturated with diluted amounts of tea tree oil are usually recommended.

A Mild Anesthetic

Tea tree oil acts as a mild anesthetic when applied to painful areas and to soothe cuts, burns, and mouth sores. It can help heal as well as reduce scarring.

Many burn victims in Australia are treated with tea tree oil. It not only helps to prevent infection and speed healing, but it also helps to soothe and relieve pain. Some of the patients received immediate relief from pain when tea tree oil was applied. Most medical professionals who deal with burn victims are extremely cautious about what they apply to the affected area. Tea tree oil may be the answer.

Help for Acne

A recent study seems to indicate the usefulness of tea tree oil in treating *acne vulgaris*. It may be used as an affective alternative to prescription medications for acne. Tea tree oil has a reputation of being gentle on the skin. It does not produce the side effects of some medications, such as dry skin, stinging, burning and slight redness after application.

Acne is most commonly seen in adolescents but may begin in childhood and continue into adulthood. It affects approximately eighty percent of the population to some degree. Lesions usually appear around puberty, and most individuals suffer from some degree of acne. It is a condition involving inflammation of the skin in the form of pimples, blackheads and whiteheads. The sebaceous glands produce oils which moisturize the skin. These glands increase in number at the onset of puberty when hormonal changes occur in the body. When the oils are blocked from entering the skin surface, irritations occur causing the acne. There may also be an increase in bacteria normally found in the glands. When a blockage occurs, inflammation may result causing a pimple.

The reason for acne is often not understood. The sebaceous glands are located in the hair follicles beneath the skin. They produce the oil that helps to moisten and lubricate the skin. When the oil is clogged in the gland, bacteria can multiply and cause inflammation or even infection. Hormonal changes may be a factor in susceptible individuals. Poor hygiene can worsen the condition when the skin surface is not kept clean.

Tea tree oil can help to heal and prevent infections from occurring. Facial cleansers, creams and lotions containing tea tree oil and the oil itself can help in preventing and treating the condition. The oil is effective in healing many types of bacteria but the most amazing thing is that is does not damage the skin tissue. Many of the recommended treatments can actually damage the skin, resulting in scarring and sensitivity. And some of the antibiotics used also destroy the beneficial bacteria needed in the body which may lead to toxicity.

A Natural Insecticide

There is no way to avoid coming into contact with insects that may bite or sting. Anyone who likes to be outdoors is vulnerable. Whether you live in the city or the country or anywhere in between, bugs abound. The most common culprits include mosquitoes, bees, gnats, fleas, spiders, ticks and ants. They can cause swelling, itching and pain. Usually, these are only an annoyance, but some are more serious. A severe allergic reaction to a bee sting or insect bite should be dealt with immediately. Black widow or brown recluse spider bites should receive emergency treatment. Deer tick bites can lead to serious conditions such as Lyme disease and Rocky Mountain Spotted Fever.

Tea tree oil can be applied to the affected area to sterilize and prevent infection. The oil also works as a anti-inflammatory to prevent and reduce swelling. It can help to neutralize the venom of insects such as wasps, bees, mosquitoes, and spiders. Insects are also known to carry different microbes such as bacteria, parasites and viruses. Tea tree oil can help stop an infection and stop the spread of the microbe if transferred to a human. The oil should be applied often and soon after the injury.

Many have used tea tree oil to counteract insect venoms. The oil is toxic to insects yet non-toxic for humans.

It is very useful for use against ticks that can carry life-threatening diseases. The oil will cause the tick to die and retract. The area should be saturated with the oil to avoid infection.

Tea tree oil or lotions and creams containing the oil can also be used to prevent bites. Insects don't like the scent of the oil and are actually repelled by it.

An Immune System Builder

The immune system in the body consists of various cells with specific responsibilities throughout the body which have the ability to recognize and destroy substances that can be harmful. The various components of the immune system try to neutralize and destroy foreign substances or infections that may invade the body. Each individual part of the immune system is unique and powerful. But they each must work together to become a match for the diseases and foreign material that may invade the body.

Some members of the immune system include white blood cells, the lymph system, immunoglobulins, interferon and interleukin. Each immune cell serves a specific function. Some know how to locate and attack antigens in the body and others must receive instructions in order to work. The white blood cells or leukocytes play a major role in fighting the battle against invaders. There are many different types and functions of the white blood cells. They are aided by other members of the immune system.

Some French physicians are studying tea tree oil for its use with the treatment of AIDS patients by strengthening the immune system of those afflicted. It is also being used to help support the immune system for individuals undergoing surgery.[15] Helping the immune system is an important element of health. The immune system is the body's defense system against anything that can cause disease or illness. Tea tree oil is a powerful immune stimulant.

Kurt Schnaubelt, Ph.D., is a leading researcher in the area of therapeutic application of essential oils. Many of his studies have reported on the ability of oils, especially tea tree oil, in stimulating immunoglobulins, known as antibodies which fight infection. "Tea Tree, Thyme and other oils are able to boost immunity by enhancing the body's own manufacture of gamma-globulin. According to one study published by essential oil researcher H. M. Gattefosse, all oils tested showed the ability to stimulate the phagocytosis to some degree."[16]

TEA TREE OIL SUPPLEMENTS

It is important to make sure that any tea tree product purchased contains only pure tea tree oil. Some synthetic products have been produced that are labeled as pure tea tree oil. The product should be wholly derived from the Melaleuca alternifolia. Other oils have been sold and labeled as pure but may contain a combination of oils. These are not as effective, Buy natural supplements from a reputable company that uses quality control measures for checking the purity of their products.

Tea tree oil can be found in many different health care products. It is in some dandruff shampoos, deodorants, toothpaste, anti-fungal ointments, anti-bacterial lotions, and in some vaginal yeast infection treatments.

USES OF TEA TREE OIL

ABRASIONS: Use a few drops of the pure tea tree oil and apply to the wound. Also use a 10 percent solution mixed with water to clean out the affected area. Use soaps containing tea tree oil to clean the area.

ACNE/PIMPLES: Apply the pure oil directly to the sore several times a day. Use a 10 percent solution and water to rinse on the face or area of pimples. Soaps can be purchases in health food stores which contain tea tree oil.

ARTHRITIS: Mix 4 to 5 drops of oil in a small amount of olive oil and massage the sore joints.

ATHLETE'S FOOT: Wash feet thoroughly with soap and water. Apply the tea tree oil directly to the feet.

BITES: For mosquito bites and bee stings dilute 1 part tea tree oil in 3 parts olive oil and apply to the affected area.

BLISTERS: Apply to the blister area twice daily. This can help heal and prevent infection.

BOILS: Use pure tea tree oil several times a day on the boil.

BURNS/SCALDS (MINOR): Dilute 1 part tea tree oil with 10 parts olive oil. Dab on the burned area.

BRUISES: Massage to bruised area twice daily.

CANKER SORES: Apply to the affected area using a cotton swab several times a day. Use at the first sign of a problem.

CHAPPED/DRY LIPS: Apply a lotion containing tea tree oil to help moisturize and heal chapped lips.

COLD SORES: Apply directly to the sore using a cotton swab. Repeat several times a day. It should stop the sore from developing.

CONGESTION: Sprinkle a few drops on a cloth and breathe through the mouth and exhale through the nose.

COUGHS/CROUP: Add pure oil to steaming water or vaporizer and inhale. Rub the oil on the chest and back.

CRADLE CAP: Mix tea tree oil with a little olive oil and rub on the scalp.

CUTS AND ABRASIONS: Apply tea tree oil directly to the cut to promote healing and prevent infection from developing.

DANDRUFF: Shampoos containing tea tree oil can help to promote a healthy scalp and normal functioning hair follicles. Rub the shampoo into the scalp and let sit for a few minutes before rinsing. A few drops of the oil can be applied directly to the scalp along with shampoo and then rinsed.

DERMATITIS: One part of tea tree oil to ten parts of cold pressed oil can be massaged into the affected areas. Tea tree soap and creams can also be useful.

DIAPER RASH: Apply to the rash by dabbing on affected areas.

DOGS/CATS: Use with shampoo when bathing the animals. It will kill lice and worms.

EAR INFECTIONS: Five drops of oil can be mixed with five drops of olive oil. Warm slightly (make sure it is not too hot) and drop a small amount into the ear.

ECZEMA: Apply tea tree oil to the area. Creams, lotions and soap containing the oil may also be useful.

FACIAL CLEANSER: Use a few drops in water and splash on face to cleanse and prevent infection.

FEET: Add 5 to 10 drops of pure tea tree oil to water and soak the feet for 5 to 10 minutes.

FUNGAL NAIL INFECTION: An undiluted solution can be applied to the nails two to three times a day.

GINGIVITIS: Rub sore gums with tea tree oil. Add a few drops to a glass of water and rinse in the mouth.

GOUT: For pain and discomfort in the joints, tea tree oil can be rubbed directly on the affected areas.

HEAD COLD: Mix ten drops of oil in a cup of hot water and inhale gently for a few minutes. It can be put in a vaporizer at night. The oil can also be rubbed under the nose.

HEAD LICE: Add ten additional drops of tea tree oil to shampoo. Massage into hair and leave on for 12 minutes, rinse and then repeat. Use at least twice a week to make sure the lice are gone.

HEMORRHOIDS: Tea tree oil can be applied directly to the area affected. A bath with ten drops of oil can be used to soothe and heal.

HIVES: Apply oil to the affected area. Lotion with tea tree oil can also be used.

INSECT BITES AND STINGS: Apply oil directly to the affected area.

INSECT REPELLENT: A combination of ten drops of oil in water can be applied to areas of the body exposed.

MOUTH SORES: Put a few drops in water and rinse mouth or apply directly to mouth sores such as canker sores to promote healing and ease pain.

MUSCLE ACHES: Add a few drops of the oil to bath water and soak or rub with olive oil on the painful areas.

NAIL INFECTIONS: Apply oil to the area affected and do not rinse off.

POISON OAK AND IVY: Massage the area with a mixture of tea tree oil and cold pressed oil. A tea tree ointment may also help.

PSORIASIS: Apply to the area affected. Lotions, creams and soaps containing tea tree oil may also be helpful.

RASHES: Apply pure oil to the affected areas to ease itching and promote healing.

RINGWORM: Apply tea tree oil directly to the area to kill the infection.

RHEUMATISM: Blend tea tree oil with cold-compressed oil and warm. Apply to painful areas as needed.

SINUS CONGESTION AND SINUSITIS: Use the pure oil in boiling water and gently inhale the vapor.

SPRAINS: Use pure tea tree oil directly on the sprain.

SORE THROAT: Add a few drops of oil to warm water and gargle twice daily as needed for pain.

SUNBURN: Add a few drops of the oil to vitamin E or aloe vera lotion. Apply a few times a day to relieve pain, redness and inflammation.

TEETHING: A solution of 1 part tea tree oil to 10 parts water can be rubbed on the gums several times a day to ease pain.

VAGINAL RINSE (INFECTIONS): Use as a douche

by adding 4 parts tea tree oil to 1,000 part water. For vaginitis it can be diluted and put on a tampon to ease discomfort and promote healing.

WARTS: Apply directly to the wart several times a day.

ENDNOTES

1 Ann Berwick. Holistic Aromatherapy. (St. Paul, MN: Llewellyn Publications, 1994), 206-207.

2 Roberta Wilson. Aromatherapy For Vibrant Health & Beauty. (Garden City, New York: Avery Publishing Group, 1995), 80.

3 Ibid., 79

4 Cynthia B. Olsen. Australian Tea Tree Oil. (Pagosa Springs, CO: Kali Press, 1991).

5 James F. Balch MD and Phyllis A. Balch, C.N.C. Prescription for Nutritional Healing. (Garden City Park, N.Y.: Avery Publishing Group Inc., 1990), 681, 682.

6 Varro E. Tyler, Ph.D. The Honest Herbal. (New York: Pharmaceutical Products Press), 307.

7 Cass Ingram, D.O. Killed On Contact. (Cedar Rapids, Iowa: Literary Visions Publishing, Inc.), 17.

8 Andrew Weil, M.D. Natural Health, Natural Medicine. (Boston: Houghton Mifflin Company), 241.

9 Cass Ingram, D.O. Killed On Contact. (Cedar Rapids, Iowa: Literary Visions Publishing, Inc.), 15.

10 Michael A. Schmidt, Lendon H. Smith and Keith W. Sehnert. Beyond Antibiotics. (Berkeley, California: North Atlantic Books), 207.

11 Tisserand R. To Heal and Tend the Body. (Wilmot, Wisconsin: Lotus Press), 1988.

12 Michael Murray, N.D. and Joseph Pizzorno, N.D. Encyclopedia of

Natural Medicine. (Rocklin, California: Prima Publishing), 532.

13 Cynthia B. Olsen. Australian Tea Tree Oil. (Pagosa Springs, CO: Kali Press, 1991) 8.

14 Cass Ingram, D.O. Killed On Contact. (Cedar Rapids, Iowa: Literary Visions Publishing, Inc.), 64-65.

15 Cass Ingram, D.O. Killed On Contact. (Cedar Rapids, Iowa: Literary Visions Publishing, Inc.), 64-65.

16 Michael A. Schmidt, Lendon H. Smith and Keith W. Sehnert. Beyond Antibiotics. (Berkeley, California: North Atlantic Books), 207.